Laurence ESTIENNE

Good-bye fibromyalgia !

How to gain twenty years and to find a good health?

Les Éditions Plum'issime

With my rebirth,

© Laurence Estienne, 2015 All rights reserved

Foreword

It would be liked that certain day is deleted of our memory. Acute pains, physical and mental sufferings which are anchored in our genetic memory.

Dubious words and little backed up speeches of the medical community, medical diagnoses unresolved, ineffective drugs which weigh on our moral. The feeling to be an object of fair and a real feeling to age prematurely in a brutal way, without the least harbinger while being insulated, being delivered to its sad fate.

The fibromyalgia imprisons you, captures you, steals you your intimacy and your dignity, bores you up to date, then constrained and subjected to deepest of your me interior to undergo its repeated attacks.

It appears without preventing, attacks part of the body, then with the other, wraps themselves, twists themselves around our being, of the head to the foot, threads with deepest of your bodies by leaving indelible traces than any doctor, neither allopathic

She imprisons us, solidifies us, returns to us dependent on her crises, a such small soldier devoted to her capricious orders. It transforms us and models us in a new envelope. Our being, a such robot, is then covered with a rigid, heavy and inflexible armour. It can be also connected with the life of an astronaut in his spacesuit. The muscles are inflated and stiffened like a wood end. The heavy and left gestures deprived of flexibility are painful. The difficulty in moving is immense. The suffering is daily. Slowness invades us. The muscular force weakens and becomes exhausted. The stretching is impossible.

Our body - until with at the time our ally becomes a source of unimaginable constraints. It is modelled like a robot whose reactions as jerked as slow and limited stick to imprison us with the ninetieth stages tree of our life. Physical comfort becomes a sad remote memory. The feeling of premature ageing of the body is immediate. The worst is than the practice must take the step on all its physical and mental sufferings. The body is accustomed and adapted then inevitably to the difficulties and incapacities. The fibromyalgia attacks at any age, in all the social layers, and indifferently of the sex and the place of residence on our beautiful terrestrial sphere. Which is this ignored, invisible, underhand evil and so powerful which steals us twenty years of your life in a quarter of second and does hostage of a destiny return to us which does no belong to us ? Within this gaol, my glance exhausted per as well sufferings escapes from day to day through the sharp-edged bars to contemplate the goal as I fixed myself to reach inaccessible star: my freedom.

Suffering from fibromyalgia for one decade, I have wish to make share my own experience through my book and bring some advices to soften his own life with the daily newspaper. I found the solution to gain twenty years and to recover a good health, my vitality and my youth.

This book is intended to the people reached of fibromyalgia, with their family and friends, their supports, with all people interested by this disease, with all the medical community which would wish to have a different vision like with the public authorities and the media, engines in the fundamental change of our French executive landscape.

First part

In the skin of another

1.

First steps

By a beautiful night of winter, in this at the beginning of January, after a few well deserved hours of deep sleep, terrible pains seize my wrist violently right. Many electric shocks imprison me and prevent me from sleeping. Massages of my front armlever cannot anything against this violent sudden and repeated attack invader. A pain without no one another similar, which launches suddenly, burns intensely at the place where it acts in my body which cannot resist the electric shocks. It is impossible to think of waiting until the pains pass in a few days. The embarrassment is so powerful and original that I promise myself to return to me in my general practitioner in the morning.

What a crowned gift the year of my forty years! I however feel young person and still full with energy.

Which body dysfunction means this evil?

From the top of my sixty-three meter, I have a fine morphology with a weight of fifty-four. I am fair with buckled long hair. I do not have anything sporting, if it is not the pace.

What a crowned gift the year of my forty years! I however feel young person and still full with energy.

Which body dysfunction means this evil? From the top of my sixty-three meter, I have a fine morphology with a weight of fifty-four. I am fair with buckled long hair. I do not have anything sporting, if it is not the pace.

A few days later, and the biological analysis in hand, the diagnosis falls on one "reassuring" muscular ignition without particular origin, apparent medical reason unresolved. The CPK and aldolase are abnormally high.

Whereas the muscular ignition quickly imprisons the integrality of my body, immobilizing my lower extremities and superiors, it is the beginning of my physical yoke!

A horror with living, supporting and to manage!

I pass by several phases in a few days: the fear tortures me. Then interrogations invade my brain. What arrives to me? Why me? What did I make to deserve that? Which is gravity? Is this the beginning of the end? How to live with? How does the disease develop? How to manage it? What will become my daughter if necessary? ... What a galley!

Despite everything, I am one beating and I do not accept my sad fate. I do not want to be sick. I think of a provisional ignition and don't give all my confidence to the medical community which hesitates, tests and seeks.

It is enough to imagine me, forty year old young woman with strong physical pains frays with an extremely reduced body mobility.

My general practitioner does not have a precise diagnosis nor of medical solution to propose to me if it is not a one week hospitalization for medical examinations. No treatment was given to me. Only time will give the medical concrete signs to cure it: one day, one week, one month, three months... Nobody knows! I remain in the most total uncertainty. A muscular biopsy should be programmed but I do not want an examination intrusive undoubtedly pulled about by a mixture of fear and pain. The option locked up at the hospital during one week for examinations does not appear accessible to me. I am then a new mother of a sixteen month old child. I do not retain it.

It is the beginning of infinite research which will last of many years to my great despair.

My pains are accentuated with the wire of the weeks and my general practitioner, conscious of this irrefutable fact, can nothing bring to me. I turn to the rheumatologist, who diagnoses a fibromyalgia and prescribes an antibiotic treatment, then considering inefficiency, an anti-inflammatory drug treatment, then paracetamol with codeine: without convincing result. I cannot believe that the fibromyalgia is a disease whose origin is unknown, which cannot be stopped nor relieved and whose impotence of the medical community is put up to date.

The months slip by in the calendar and the pains always resist and make my body a zombie because he does not answer my requests any more since too long. In fact, my hope of a provisional ignition starts to be reduced. Do I have to be made with the idea be sick with life? In a few months, my resistance is reduced. My dynamism flies away giving way to a slowness and especially with deep limitations of the whole of my movements.

In addition to my great difficulty of driving me, like a mammoth with its heaviness, its slowness and its sinistrality, my spirit, as for him, are slowed down, at the same time obnubilated by my health problems worsened and anxious of the future that they hold for me.

Tiredness was right of my social life, family and professional. At the end of one year of tiredness, I became exhausted physically. My mother however alerted me often on my weight loss but I refused to hear it. I waited of the better days. I saw myself different from the glance of the other. However, I was frightened by my spectacular weight loss. In four months, I had the feeling to play jackpot of the kilos. And one, two, three, and four kilos in less! Five, six, seven, eight!!! I then lost ten kilos! My older brother, teaser at his hours, even compared to me, in his great kindness, in "Auschwitz". With his departure, I cried all the tears of my body. I had indeed only the skin on my bones. The bones of my basin bored at sight of eye my skin, the necklace of bone around my neck was accentuated, my face was emaciated, my cheeks grew hollow, my arms resembled to an articulated puppet... The whole accentuated by a spectacular muscular cast iron. My forty-four kilos carried me towards an irreversible physical decline if I were not caught charges some quickly. In spite of my obstinacy nothing to be seen, I had the feeling to have a silhouette of mannequin! I wanted at the same time to protect my family from my physical disorders and strove to hide the sad truth to them, while consolidating me in the almost immature hope of better days where my health would take again the top.

I thus went in my new general practitioner in January to alert it of my descent into Hell then in April to ask him to help me because I could not only arrive there any more. How it is difficult to ask of the assistance! But the urgency was such as I could not make differently. I felt impotent. I did not have any more the force to react. I did not know the emergency exit. I did not feel courageous. I lost my forces. I did not manage to guide my life of adult suitably as I always did. I was mother and responsible for my offspring. I was to raise me and cope. But how? No doctor understood my distress. No concrete solution was brought to me. Well sometimes my mother gave me remains of cooked dishes. Transformed into object of curiosity, except standards, my health status was incomprehensible for the common run of people. And yet, quite real for me which lived it with each breathing!

What would it have been necessary in these moments of loneliness? The physical pain is immense, abyssal even! Insulation, loneliness, the feeling to be single in its corner, the feeling not to have any exit door, to have missed my life, to find me at the bottom of the hole, not to advance, come very close to opposition to progress, not to benefit from the life, not to be understood, to be used for nothing, to be old and ugly, to be useless and scraggy, to be a pit and a waste for the company! So many negative thoughts invaded my head. My spirit nothing any more but seemed blocked by this crowned disease. Each gesture brought back to me to it. Each second I lived through it.

My general practitioner, initially reticent with cortisone, true balsam for the body which hides a development of an unspecified disorder, finally decided to prescribe it (during four years of thirty milligrams per day the first month then twenty-five milligrams for three months, until a progressive reduction two last years with two milligrams). Lacteous drinks very proteins by regular cure were prescribed to me. This food mode was saving. The pains were clearly reduced and my weight started to be packed. In six months, I found my silhouette of yesteryear. Other seals against the anxiety, muscular relaxation, and the vitamin D were added. My muscular diminish and tendinitises remained in the state, preventing me progressing favorably and from gaining in flexibility. The important profit was that of the progression of the disease stopped thanks to cortisone, and the clear reduction in the pain while preserving the intact state of strong diminish. I cannot go beyond my diminish and I do not feel a pain. This was a great relief for me. How to live this painful state at the same time in my forty year old head and the body of a ninety year old woman?

From where can the real origin come from my evils? I do not want to be locked up in this black circle. The years pass and I refuse to be sick. I do not believe in it. I wonder during long hours about their origin. I want to leave my search with convincing elements. With the wire of my reflections in search of coïncidentes, I go back to my childhood and course again the way of my life on a medical, sentimental and professional level. I seek the repetitions, the big events, happy or unhappy of my life. I draw from my memory. I do a long research task on my family during several months.

2.

Postural and physical disorders

I feel blocked, stiffenet, prevented by a supernatural force from carrying out all the simple gestures of the life. I take little by little possession of an armour as a body. My muscles and tendons inflated, stiffened by the muscular ignition. They prevent any classical movement and any mobility. My feet are then at light-years of my hands!

1 - Postural disorders

Loss of body flexibility

More far from my memory, my body was always flexible. With the college or the high school, I liked to make the straight shaft or the wheel. I often stretched myself and I had a feeling of wellness in this state. I had leaning for the PE on the ground. However, year by year imperceptibly, I stiffened, without same giving me an account of it. At twenty years, at the time of the rocker before my bust to lean me, legs tended to reach the ground with my fingers tended arms, I did not manage any more to pose my hands flat on the ground. During a trip to Rome with my parents, at the twenty years age, I remember one day of intense walk for visits of monuments. I felt my muscles to stiffen with the hollow of the knees during the night. With the rising, I had lost any mobility! I felt strong stiffnesses and had difficulty walking quickly to follow the steps of my family. Undoubtedly, the origin is the heating of my muscles by a on-request. That resulted in a painful feeling of burn to walk, especially the cold muscle.

Then a few years later, to touch the point of the fingers on the ground tended legs, I was to draw on my back inordinately.
To about thirty, I practised the tennis shoe equips senior with it during two seasons. I adored this sport with the college. I was captain of team. My professor of sport had noticed me and even proposed to return in the departmental team. I was voluntary, fast, and always at the head vis-a-vis the opposing team to mark shopping carts and to however mobilize my adversaries towards the victory, I choked with each crossing of ground while running. My endurance was at the minimum level. I became red scarlet at the end of the match. I was not at ease to run quite simply. My vitality and my physical dynamism were reduced.

I took courses of bar on the ground at thirty-seven years which made me become aware that my youth moved away. Sat on the ground, drawn aside legs, of large dorsal stiffnesses prevented my projection ahead. My fingers had much difficulty of catching my feet! My stiffened thighs could not be spread out when I leaned my bust on each leg. In addition to the time which passes, I was well blocked by an invisible force which retained me inordinately.

Problem of posture

The feeling to leave on the right side while going is usual. The lack of stability is obvious. My steps are light, seeking to compensate for it. My arch of the foot does not bring a catch on the ground sure and firm. I understood eight years later the origin of this dysfunction.

2 - Body disorders

The body

To understand quickly that impossibility of lowering me ahead or of beign squatted, with great difficulties to sit me and of raising me of a chair because of strong muscular tensions which numb my thighs belonged to my daily newspaper. To sleep flat belly is not possible any more.

The rise and the descent of the steps are complicated to apprehend, only one after the other, as the infants do it.

Prolonged walk is to be avoided because it causes crispations on the level of the thighs, calves, neck and shoulders. It is even impossible in rough or even stony ground.

Kitchen, the maintenance of the house (to pass the vacuum cleaner, the floorcloth, to press a sponge, to make the beds...), the races (handling of the articles and their weight), to lead or to occupy me of my family life with an young child with load (daily care) are a drudgery and from now on to make with precaution and slowly.

My daughter with the crib feeds normally at midday while I buy manufactured goods to nourish me with work.

Top of the body

The posture changes on the level of the ahead posted stiffened neck and the shoulders without being able to turn on both sides completely.

Members

My members are stiff like stakes with a great difficulty of raising my arms. To close a bra with the arms in the back became impossible to me.

Many night alarm clocks strew my nights. Pains paralyse me the upper limbs and lower. Because of prolonged positions of the legs and folded arms, the least movement of deployment of my legs and my arms fights on my stiffened muscles thus requested. What a pain! Obligation to move if not remain ankylosed me accompanied forever by a sharp feeling of burn in my muscles with my very slow movement on my hard and stiff articulations. It was terrible with living and so painful.

Skin

A hard-bound skin, dry and irritated on all the body is added, badly irrigated, of a bluish and marbled color.

The face

Oral wrinkles

In rise from the oral wrinkles, broad band vertical around the mouth which accentuates already premature ageing by the disease.

Oral contracting

It followed quickly with an opening to only two centimeters and half.

Stretching of the skin

Especially on the face on the level of the face and the mouth, the excessive stretching of the skin works an unaesthetic mask.

Mouth

I have a feeling of tinglings inside my cheeks and especially on my language with having to eliminate the toothpaste with mint when I wash myself the teeth. To chew a chewing-gum with mint is not desirable.

Hands

The most awkward phenomenon is the impossibility of closing/opening of the hands with loss of force. Driving of a car was difficult but not insurmountable for me, the paper ranking, the writing or the striking of awkward documents but not prohibited... The paper handling is extremely reduced and causes cracks quickly. The hands flat are not possible any more. The articulations are red.

It is enough to imagine a permanent opening of the hands with almost tended, slightly curled up and deformed fingers! Covers become difficult to hold, the knife to be wristd, the heavy kitchen utensils to carry, glasses well too broad for my new morphology... The sensitivity of the skin to the level of the end of the fingers is extremely fine. Gripping is consequently awkward and painful. To feel its last phalange is handicapping and invalidating.

An undeniable loss of force and an impossibility are closely dependent to carry weight (flour, a bottle, a water bottle, a frying pan... A signature book with work is heavy and its transport is done on my front armlevers. Just like to raise my daughter to raise it of her bed the morning or after the nap is a meticulous operation with my front armlevers. She slept in a bed of "large" made safe by a barrier.

The arrival of the dead hand, on the level of the hands - whose cold numbs and bleaches the ends obliges to have on oneself gloves and to avoid in the supermarkets their fresh and frozen rays.

Clothing

In order to avoid any complication, it is usual to equip me differently, to fit me differently, (without lace), more not to put a too heavy, too hard on the skin and too cumbersome jewelry, and to forget the rings which wound between the fingers by their friction.

Difficulty of motricity

A great difficulty of moving invaded me. The impression to be in the body of another obsessed me. I am identified with a young person in the body of an old person. My cramp generalized led to an incapacity to release me. I do not manage to have any muscular relaxation. For about ten year, my body has become foreign and behaves with its own way. I do not recognize it any more. He does not answer my requests any more. I differently without request it to be able to release it, alleviate it, relieve it.

It is compressed, oppressed, and tended. The cold accentuates this phenomenon. It is my capital, I must however take care and give preferential treatment to it of it.

Increased fatigability: 40% of my life to sleep

The evening as if one had given me a blow of bludgeon on skull, I fell asleep at a stretch, in front of the TV with twenty-and-a hour thirty at the latest. I did not derogate from this rule. I kept this rhythm since my adolescence, faithful to this principle. Not an evening, I could look at a film in his entirety! My memories of schoolgirl bring back for me to the parental authorization on television to look at all the tuesday evening the western on one of the three chains possible. Systematically, I slept of a heavy and major sleep and the next morning, I found myself in my bed, in which my father had deposited me the day before at the end of the film. Adult, I continued this ritual. I can say that I consumed televisual films of them! Every evening, I hamper in front of the small screen. My eyes became so heavy that I could not fight. The sleep is stronger than all, it carried me in its wake. Chronic tiredness is a plague, a curse, a handicap. To take care the evening was always very uncomfortable to me. This lack of vitality seized me at the bottom of my entrails without being able to fight. After me to be awaked at twenty-two hours thirty, after the famous film which should have held me in breath, I returned in my bed carried very quickly in a night of torpor, without feeling of dreamed, until the morning. At seven hours, awaked by the ringing of the cicadas of my morning alarm clock, I rise, with to have slept the well feeling. My vital need of a long night of sleep accounted for nine to ten hours of sleep. To tell the truth, at forty years, I slept forty-two percent of my life!

Lack of energy

Such an amount of diminish and of stiffnesses the body weakens. Energy flies away forever. My lack of energy was obvious. I am deprived of any will. The least action seems to me a mountain to be crossed. All becomes insurmountable. My body is unsuited to the effort and prevented any activity.

Slimming

Physical tiredness involves moral tiredness and an inevitable slimming that it is good to suppress. However, I fell into this vicious circle with a loss ten kilos. The doctors know this phenomenon but do not anticipate. The muscular cast iron is source of evils and physical difficulties of which it is all the more hard to cope. Months even of the years are necessary to go up the slope.

Reluctance

Since my most remote memory, I always suffered from reluctance. My blood circulation seems disturbed. What a unpleasant feeling the sensitive to cold ones are confronted! The least air, even summer, is uncomfortable and unpleasant for me. It transforms me into ice floe of the head to the foot. My ends solidify instantaneously. My nose, my hands, and my feet are fresh even cold. Impossible to heat me without an additional thickness. I always take care to have a sweater close to me, of the fine gloves in my bag as well as a light bonnet.

Disorders of mood

The body tensions involve a lack of control in my reactions.

Receptive with the atmospheric pressure

In rainy or windy weather, my body reacts in an unfavourable way. It is charged with negative ions which disturb the diminish and support the cracks and the drought of the skin.

The list is not exhaustive because the daily newspaper in general weighs heavy and poses problem. At every moment, my slow and awkward gestures bring back for me to painful reality. I am prevented. I am stiff head with the foot.

3 - Medical care and surgical

Preventive cure

In addition, in order to mitigate the nuisances of the infantile diseases, the pediatrist had taken to us as guinea-pigs, my older brother and myself with in nursery school and primary education to try out a preventive cure of injections of gamma globulin to spend the winter. The nurse made us very painful punctures in the buttocks. The pain was intense and its memory as much. My cries at the time as of punctures of the nurse, the feeling to undergo in the constraint, without understanding of it the pseudonyms benefits, the absence of my mother who did not support to see and to hear and the imposing presence of my father seemed to me a torture. Of this episode, I hedge punctures in all its forms, of the blood tests to acupuncture with me to feel some badly, to contract me and to even have a discomfort when the nurse disastrous. While not being sick, I was in an infernal spiral of medical constraints without which I would have readily done. My mistrust near the medical community was already on the way. It proved that this pediatrist was suspended of his functions during three years, in the end of a career for illicit exercise of medicine.

Oral problems

I tested very young person the experiment of the dentist and the decays. From the top of my six years, my decays developed, with one, on a tooth then another, bound for a premolar receptive whose enamel was friable. In the Seventies, the dentist did not use water with the caster. Of my memories of childhood, it turned slowly but got pains to me and had a smell of burning. I did not love the dentist. Why decays? However, I did not eat a candy, nor did not drink sweetened juices. Undoubtedly that my final teeth were weakened by the absorption of "tétracycline", drug prescribes at the three years age to look after my whooping-cough. For a few years, this drug has been interdict with the children of less than eight years! It was recognized that the teeth undergo the devastating effect of this antibiotic. It weakens the teeth by friable e-mail on the final teeth in preparation and dyes of an abnormal coloring the final teeth in an irreversible way of a darker gray towards the gum which is degraded of a tone more clearly downwards. I already undergo with my young age the effects of the medical inconsistencies: the public health which puts on the market bound for the young children of the unsuited drugs. My baby teeth, white like pearls, were replaced by final teeth tried and striated with unpleasant let us tons of darker gray degraded towards the gum on the integrality of my teeth.

I tried to make a whitening of teeth by gutters in my dentist in 1995 - not refunded by the social security on the lower and higher incisors. The result was convincing because I recovered two colors but the gray persists still nowadays. Fear to make the teeth more fragile slows down me in the realization of other gutters twenty years afterwards. The retreat is not made on this kind of symptoms contrary to the color by drinks (coffee, tea) or cigarettes.

Alleviating recommendation is made to me by my dentist to about thirsty especially not chew a chewing-gum because of large amalgams which could not resist the pressure, to make salivate while increasing the dental risk of break.

Great difficulties in opening my jaw only tighten to the maximum the tendons of the contour of the mouth for an opening of two centimeters. To bite an apple becomes very complicated and painful like a burn.

Operation of appendicitis

At the nine years, I was operated of an appendicitis attack which pulled about me since long months to more be able to go lengthily. Market day, I was to have breaks to return on foot to the house. The abdominal pains drew me in the low belly to more be able to take a step. The only solution was the forced rest and the reclining position during thirty minutes. This test with the so young private clinic does not leave me indifferent. First general anaesthesia with drowsiness with the balloon to avoid the punctures for which I have a holy horror of it, then the irresistible desire to drink after my alarm clock without having the possibility of it, the difficulty in going the following day with abdominal pain, the first night out of my cocoon family, in a hostile world, accompanied by my cuddly toy, a large tried white rabbit of beige offered by my parents and the memory of a meal jumped by lapse of memory of the nurse. My appendicitis in a transparent tube was ignited and blackened and not was very pretty to see after the operation. Its memory is very present still. My scar is almost invisible and I must rent competences of the surgeon.

Affections face

Chronic sinusitises, rhinitides are the object of my daily newspaper since the Nineties. I suffered from colds, of nose stopped with repetition without to catch cold. I consulted a specialist who indicated to me that my nasal partition was deformed a little but that nothing justified these repetitions. He recommended a nasal spray with each crisis. I used of the tons of handkerchiefs paper during years. Release generally takes place in spring what could make think of an allergic origin.

Voltage drop

I become exhausted regularly. With each change of season, my tension approaches the nine and of the flies have fun to pass in front of my eyes with difficulties of descending the staircases and a strange feeling to have my cotton legs a such headstock of rag. The fear of falling without being able to retain me and of breaking me a member considering their extreme stiffnesses to be yielded pulls about me. It is the sign of a well deserved rest.

Vaccination with the mode

I had to protect me from the diseases. The vaccines had the good share on my body against the infantile diseases. I also tested at thirty years the vaccine of hepatitis B stopped in the course of treatment (three catches) considering the side-effects disparaged by the public opinion.

Three months before my muscular ignition, I had the vaccine of the DT polio. One knows the interrogations mitigated on the fatal consequences of the vaccines on the human body and the release of diseases.

Dermatological problems

Quickly, the strong ones diminish, the limitation of the movements and the lack of sport reduced the blood circulation causing of the problems of skin to the level of the hands with cracks and the over-sensitiveness of the ends of the fingers. The drought on the level of the hands is important. The skin is hard-bound on the level of the front armlevers. The color is bluish. Itchings seem to relieve the drought close to the wrists. The articulations are red. The fingers on the level of the phalanges and the articulations are inflated. The cuticles are non-existent. Certain nails are striated. The nails are almost white with the tended fingers. The phalanges are red.

No dermatologist, general practitioner, or pharmacist could not bring to me an effective solution for the relief of the drought to the level of the palm of the hands and especially of the fingers. I test all the creams marketing! Moreover, of the small buttons appeared in the palms of the hands from time to time.

My body also presents signs of drought on the legs (especially calves and feet) and the arms.

In 2011, my problems of skin on the level as of hands are unbearables. For four long years I have not seen improvement. I hope for some advices by another medical community.

Exceptionally, the dermatologist, department head of the hospital, grant a hospitalization of day to me over two days close to my place of dwelling for some medical examinations. Direction the ophthalmologist which, after a torture and retina to see the state of my eyes and to estimate if a drug (with side-effect: an ocular attack) could be to me prescribed. The drug is abandoned because not very advanced state of the disease. Ocular torture could have been avoided!

Pulmonary attack

In 2011, only a small alveolar pulmonary attack is discovered. Examinations on my pulmonary capacity are carried out and confirm a respiratory restriction of 30% compared to a woman of my age. The pulmonary fibrosis is to be supervised each year. It will have been necessary to wait five years to make this examination and this observation!

Problem of immunity

It is auto-immune question also of disease: the syndrome of overlapping of scleroderma and the "dermatomyosite" considering the physical symptoms.

The antinuclear antibodies 1/800 and anti PMScl are positive this year, that is to say five years after the muscular ignition. The medical community puts finally a name on the disease: scleroderma. She belongs to the orphan diseases (a weak part of the population is reached by it) although she spreads herself more and more near the women nowadays.

It is true that to know of which affection one suffers, relieves our mental. One knows with what to better expect. In fact, it is about a not very widespread pathology. It can attack the vital bodies what is not my case. It is right at the first stage and has not evolved for ten years. That strongly encourages me to gain day in day the combat against it.

Appearance of nodules

In 2011, after the end of the cortisone catch, of the nodules under cutaneous appeared on my articulations of the elbows and the knees especially. Impossibility of making a taking away by the dermatologist considering the attachment with the tendons did not make it possible to determine their invisible composition because with the radio (whereas they could have been calcification).

4 - Deteriorated quality of life

My life in general was disturbed by all these failures and all these difficulties what resulted in a clear reduction in my physical performances. The vital minimum was necessary and the rest necessary to each moment of freedom out of professional framework.

I lost autonomy with the direction clean of the term i.e. feasibility to carry out an unspecified task with facility. Great difficulties with loss of landmarks plunged me following my muscular ignition in a deep distress which cannot be understood by the common run of people if it is not that which lives this situation with the identical one. All appears insurmountable to me.

Great difficulties to use my daily retracted hands slow down me in the integrality of my movements and return me a degraded, out-of-date and unbearable image of my own person. I took twenty, even fifty years at a stretch! I am in a body of a person of the old aged while preserving my youth mental of my forty years ! I suffer in my stiff body like a robot, imprisoned in an armour, without same power to stretch me. The daily newspaper quickly becomes a source of frustrations.

Loss of autonomy in the domestic activities

I feel captive of my body. I lose my reference marks. I have as well difficulties to make as to manage the house, the kitchen (to peel, cut, carry the kitchen utensils) and maintenance (brush, floorcloth, dust) very complicated and are carried out with pain and burns.

Loss of autonomy in the social activities and leisures

The desire flew away for leaving at home because all appears insurmountable to me. I apprehend the only fact of moving my body! The leisures pass from now on to the second plan. With work, the pain is added to my gestural slow and difficult. I am constantly prevented in my simplest movements of the daily newspaper: to take compound of the telephone, to make fresh starts of a file, to write, sit me, raise me, lower me, recover an object on the ground...

Loss of autonomy in family

My difficulty of occupying me of my daughter in low age however gave me the force to overcome my difficulties, obliged to raise it and meet its needs. This enabled me not to ankylose and to develop more force on my right hand because I am right-handed.

Loss of autonomy in the personal care

The first difficulty is to take a bath. The sitting position on the ground is impossible for me unless dropping me on the buttocks. But how to make to raise me with my hands in form of hook, without force and mobility? To take the shower in the bath-tub is a difficult martyrdom because of access without being able to raise the posts which are used to me as legs. To stabilize itself then on a slipping ground concerns the exploit. Much precautions and time are necessary.

How the ground is low! My feet are well far from my hands! What a difficulty to fit to me, put sticking or of the socks, to cut me nails and to put varnish to me, and to even wash me feet!

The back is also a difficult zone of access. That to say my face which never seemed to me to be also osseous with my hooked fingers which cannot apprehend it easily. To extend a cream on the body of the end of the fingers - with pain in the torsion of the wrist and stiffnesses in the fingers is rich lesson.

3.

Digestive disorders

Vomiting with repetition

Since my more young age, I frequently had acetone crisis and bilious attacks until adolescence. My speciality was the vomiting in spite of me! Memories of evil being due to the evils of belly, from bitterness in the mouth, burn in the stomach, tiredness… return. Transport accentuated this phenomenon. Then came the period from intestines disfonctionnements to repetition each year during about twenty years.

Inopportune distensions

Since my more tender childhood, I suffered from distensions with repetition. It is the symptom which characterizes me more. One can think a little girl with a belly inflated like a goldbeater's skin! Weakened by fizzy drinks, dairy produces and the wheat flour, my intestines were made the good share show their existence with the common run of people. Shame tortured me. With the sea, with my two-piece swimsuit, and my fine and slim silhouette, I raised a round belly good tended like the Biafran ones of the third world in Africa. My clothes were limited to sizes above mine, (one to two) of broad, full clothing to hide my repetitive swellings. I even tested at twenty years the maternity garments with pants which, resolutely, were not adapted to my fine morphology.

These distensions took to me at any hour of the day, without generally preventing accompanied by pains before thirty years and important intestinal disorders after this age. Often quickly after the meal, with a pasta dish with the tomatoes, crudenesses, a consumption of factory-baked bread, milk, fizzy drinks, I was a collector of intestines problems and distensions. Discomfort was there. I thought a long time that the raw food was responsible. It was my second brain! It without any doubt reacted to the daily pressure, too strong to swallow by my true brain. Hypersensitive and secret, I had difficulty hiding my emotions through my belly. It inflated air, as to tell me that it had some enjoys. Over the years, it was to support the lowering of any food in fast meals, the stress of work, the vibrating life of the race job-sleep. It thought of my place... So many false excuses which did not give any improvement as for their suppression in my everyday life.

My problems of intestines were never diagnosed by a general doctor and specialist. No specific drug nor no council was given to me to cure it. I consulted a no officially agreed general doctor in the years 2000 which spoke to me for the first time the probiotics ones to consume in cure. Thanks to their absorption, the improvement was made feel in my organization without to evacuate the less frequent disadvantages. However, I recently almost eliminated milk and his derivatives and reduces my gluten consumption (manufactured good, bread, products sweetened...) My digestive comfort improved inevitably without in a spectacular way.

4.

Cognitive disorders

1 - Lower intellectual performances

The heaviness of the disease involves the fall of all in particular intellectual capacities. The mental one does not follow any more because obsessed by the evil and subjected to insulation. The brain is softened sclerosed, emptied. I passed from administrative competitions during many years without having a sufficiently positive result in spite of my professional competences and my level of studies. I have the feeling to be beside my shoes.

Memory loss

I have had a facility of training and a good memory for my young school years. My visual memory helps me much. However, in addition to the weight of the ages which limits the memory, I could note a certain difficulty of memorizing.

Difficulty of attention

My concentration at every moment on my evil with the alarm clock of each pain me prevented from having a continuous concentration. I live my evil at each second because he recalls me systematically with his memory.

2 - Field of the emotions and the sensitivity

Anxiety :

The confrontation of the disease in a dubious future worries our unconscious and uses our daily newspaper. The physical pains are added with the mental pains and form a cocktail which weakens us. The doctors cannot treat that by tranquillizers - provisional buoy of help and even prescribe antidepressants which relieve only of the symptoms and mask reality. The life is unbearable in the suffering but it is it of as much with my direction that food with antidepressants.

Perception

Simple sight of a heavy or difficult object of handling (like the stopper of a pen or a water bottle) or the volume of load to be carried out (like the paper sorting, the fact of dividing into sheets a magazine...) disturb me with the fear not there of not arriving and of having to use of the physical force which I lost.

Memory loss

I have had a facility of training and a good memory for my young school years. My visual memory helps me much. However, in addition to the weight of the ages which limits the memory, I could note a certain difficulty of memorizing.

Difficulty of attention

My concentration at every moment on my evil with the alarm clock of each pain me prevented from having a continuous concentration. I live my evil at each second because he recalls me systematically with his memory.

Second part

Comforts of life

Last chaos and these months of "zombie", in the skin of another, I awoke with the firm will of me to leave there. I could not convince me that I was sick. I did not deserve that. I had always had a calm and healthy life without excess. What would thus have started this disease?

1.

The medical shutter

1 – allopathic medicine

I never had great confidence with the medical community. At five years, the only pediatrist, recommended a mode containing punctures month containing "gamma-globuline" in order to prevent the extremely painful infantile diseases. This treatment however was not effective since my brother and myself naps not reached of auto-immune disease. The trauma of the punctures still remains intact and engraved in my memory. I apprehend the least needle and the blood tests are for me a martyrdom. I stiffen all my body with the sight of a simple needle. For as much, I hopelessly search a certain comfort of life to reduce my stiffnesses.

Vaccination

The modification of procedure of vaccination of hepatitis B by the public authorities still questions me. Some agree to say that aluminium in the vaccines could disturb immunity and develop autoimmune diseases. But the benefit of the vaccines being more important than the possible problems, the vaccines remain on the market.

The vaccination of the DT Polio three months before my muscular ignition returns to me perplexed even if the doctors grant themselves to say that the retreat is sufficiently large not to overpower it.

Meetings of kinesitherapy

Three meetings of physio per week bring to my body the benefits of easing and wellness to the level of the neck, the back, the legs and the hands. Lymphatic drainage of the lower extremities and superiors give me a feeling of lightness in my arms and my legs. I tested many physios. Some are turned towards the relaxation and relieving with soft massages, others make useful massages (hands, feet, back). The benefit is always present.

Hospital medical controls

In order to improve my daily newspaper, I turned to the University hospital to in 2011 be followed regularly by same staffs and identical equipment.

Examinations were carried out and it could be carried out an annual medical monitoring. No unfavourable evolution since 2011. However, the feeling to be an object of curiosity during consultations of the interns and visits of students is rather strong and rather unpleasant in front of the empty glance of medical staff and the absence of comment.

Over the years since the muscular ignition, it was indicated to me by the medical community the following successive diseases: the fibromyalgia, the "dermatomyosite", the syndrome of overlapping scleroderma and "dermatomyosite" then scleroderma following the positive marker of the antibodies. It is to say that the diagnosis was dubious during five years, period during which I made only regular blood tests.

Therapeutist in body ergonomics

My meeting with the therapeutist of the hospital put to me balsam in the middle thanks to its optimism and with its competences. Large curly brown woman with the sharp glance which combines its professional competences with its empathy, its direction of the communication and its good mood. With each one of my meetings, I gain a few millimeters in the opening and the closing of my hands. She works on the "fascias" which are fine membranes which wrap the muscles and bodies which contract in particular on crispations, the stress and gets manual massages which facilitate the work of relaxation of the tendons. Helped of tools powerful, it makes me work three hours per day during one week. The mental one must be accustomed to gain in flexibility and to find postures which it does not integrate any more. Work per moment gives the impression which the fingers will break because of the apprehension and of the pain but the profit is certain: one half-centimeter per finger per week. The meetings are tiring but so beneficial. For as much, work is done carefully, with massages and adequate handling with pathology. I gained three centimeters per finger with closing thanks to his intervention in four cures. My objective remains the total closure of my hands. The articular amplitude not being reached, the hope is not a lure. The disadvantage of the trade is its assumption of responsibility a year according to strict rules of hospitalization at a rate of two to three times. The occupational therapy is useful for the improvement of the symptoms even to their cure. This speciality is not developed enough in our country.

2 - Alternative medicines and parallel

Benefits of yoga and the sophrology

I practised during two years hastened it yoga in the Eighties, taught by a woman of experiment. The movements slow and applied easing and of stretching, maintenance and force bring a comfortable wellness mental physics and, relieving and a plenitude as well as a body tonicity. This one hour daily complete physical practice thirty minutes brings such a mental relaxation that is set up a Zen attitude which lasts a few days even the week. Many benefits are recognized in this technique from India. But since my health problems, it is impossible for me to put to me on the ground. However, I practise abdominal breathing in order to alleviate me.

Analysis of the genealogy

That was the occasion to make research on my genealogy and to build my family tree in order to understand my family tree in order to understand my family history. I invite even my ancestors to my course in order to find the links between the beings and their similarities. Helped of the birth dates as of the my ancestors and their course of life, I made interesting discoveries. I annotate genetic criteria, identifications, resemblances, a family fidelity, etc I manage little by little to establish links. On my coloured pallet the structured features of my programmed history take shape then.

Meetings of kinesiology

The kinesiologist, former nurse, practises the kinesiology, with several techniques since long years. Lengthened on a bed, I let myself go to the relaxation. It uses the pendulum, the stones, essential oils, the cards of the plants. She questions space time (present, last, future) with the pendulum in order to leave in search of a possible dysfunction.

It emphasized my weaknesses, my fears and my interrogations. I spoke to him about my professional blockings. It enabled me to pose a positive image on myself for going from the front one. As of the first meeting, I could note the benefit of work on energies because I became aware of my competences of writer and the result of my project of writing of book about ten days afterwards. I then created my structure of public letter-writer "Plum' issime". She asked me as often as possible to put a precise image of plant in my crossing points in order to have it with the sight. Arrived at my residence, I took my brushes and I painted the flowered image. This first meeting was very profitable because it developed my creativity. Two other meetings followed. The kinesiologist at the same time surprised and was charmed benefit of his actions. She indicated to me that I will remain in his annals.

Magnetism

Tested approximately fifteen years before for problems of professional overwork and tiredness, I turned to a hypnotizer. I leave these meetings with an energy and a relaxation which do much good to me. I return there to reload me in energy and to alleviate my tensions. I am very satisfied with this practice.

The discovery of acupuncture

I also turned to acupuncture which enabled me to make circulate energies in my body. With each weekly session, the needles planted in the back, the shoulders, the top of skull and the ears perforated my body whose fine skin generally felt the punctures like physical aggressions. An evil for a good because in my calves circulated an uninterrupted flood of boiling, a such torrent.

The discovery of homeopathy

I decided to consult a homeopath for a basic work, on the immunizing ground. A homeopath more incites me to invest me in a long-term treatment because the number of amounts is tiny room to only one treatment at the same time against various tubes with a classical homeopath. But the notoriety of the classical homeopath leaned in the balance.

The homeopathic treatment in the long run and a processing against prevention flu were given to me.

Recently, I went to consult a homeopath in my area removes the allergies. Equipped with small flasks containing the allergens, it deposits each flask selected on my neck (while being lengthened) then, by a simple pressure on the level as of temples, it tests the allergy. Then, without physical contact, it removes the problem. It found me an allergy to lead, mercury, the BCG and arsenic. I had to note that my morning loose cough clearly attenuated as of the following day. At the time of my second consultation, following the demounting of my last crown, it found me an allergy to mercury, lead, the hays and dust, the environmental allergies, vaccine ROR and the gamma rays. Twice, it had to test the mercury and the lead which seem anchored well to deepest of my bodies. I felt the immediate effects in my legs at the moment when the flask is deposited on my neck. Rare are the people who perceive this sensitivity. He added another product without me to reveal the name of it in order to note the effects. I felt tinglings of the feet to the head, as a current which traversed me all the body with shivers per moments when the pressure is too strong, then a strong pressure on skull (at the base and the top of the head especially), for then escaping by the seventh will chakra.

The benefit on cough is even more obvious and the drought of the hands improved.

The discovery of osteopathy

After the birth of my daughter, meetings of osteopathy brought an appreciable comfort to me because my body was not in its axis. My basin bored ahead on the right. In position upright, my body leans on before my feet. My toes support the entirety of the weight thus. My basin leaves ahead, my back grows hollow, my shoulders arch slightly and my neck compensates for the position behind. The correction of the osteopath to each one of my visits brings a body lightness to me which makes good with the body and the moral one.

Relaxation by heat and the massages

I began from the meetings of massage on my ravaged body by so much of muscular tensions. My stiffnesses could not support any change such as walk on foot prolonged, race, bicycle, yoga and sophrology (impossible to put to me on the ground), swimming pool (premature draining of the skin and especially of the hands with cracks)... A little softness on my skin proves to have a relaxing, resting effect, releasing, and even relieving congestion. A few minutes of wellness compared with hours of tensions! The massage with the hot stones facilitated my physical increase vis-a-vis months of exhaustion and pain. My budget is burdened with meetings of massages in various places.

I in addition took a subscription for weekly sessions of balneotherapy. This one hour meeting brings an insane good to me. Heat is appropriate to me perfectly. The relaxation brought by this kind of technique followed by a tea gets a total happiness to me.

Plantar reflexology

On several occasions, I profited from the plantar benefits of massages. The points of acupuncture, the meridian lines and the centers of our energies on the surface of the foot help circulation to be propagated in all the body. The result is surprising. A total relaxation wraps us, the foot is light and flexible walk.

3 - Improvement of my food

Considering the intestinal disorders and distensions, I have turned to a change of food for one year.

Wheat flour

The wheat flour evolved to the detriment of its quality. The gluten ingurgitation in the body goes against the wellness digestive. It is important to wonder about the need for eating cooked bread or dishes. I for my part removed most of food containing wheat flour and my intestines feel much better.

Dairy produces

I tested the food without dairy produces. I stopped drinking chocolate milk. I avoided yoghurts during a few months. I could note a thinning at the abdominal level and a digestive comfort. It is true that in the Seventies, the yoghurts were sold with the unit in a container out of glass. Today, the trade on large scales transformed the yoghurt consumption to the detriment of nutritional quality.

The research of the defense of immunity

In the year 2005, I made the meeting of a general practitioner except nomenclature which recommended the probiotics ones. Still ignored at the time, I however took his advice. I made cures lasting of the months in order to improve my transit and to find good intestines. Recently, on the advices of a pharmacist, I moved towards a general doctor who, through very detailed biological analyses carried out in Belgium. One month after, the results except standards are seized in the adequate software of the doctor who concludes with a homeopathic treatment to order in a specialized laboratory in Belgium. The long-term treatment consists of amounts with 1000K and mixtures of granules specific to dilute in a little bottle of water with catch day labourer of a small spoon.

In order to preserve a relative autonomy, the research of the functionality is required to have a maximum of comfort, of security and effectiveness in its gestures. To put all the chances of cure on its side, it is important to be active, to stop smoking and to have a balanced food.

2.

Advices and tips

The worst in the disease is to let itself deal with by medicine, to put themselves instead of "patient" and to let themselves guide by the doctor without anything to make. Because the disease guides our steps. It is easy to return in its slippers and to wait better days. This passive attitude vis-a-vis the life is harmful for survival. The advices of the general practitioner are rare in order to improve his hygiene of life by medicine.

In order to preserve a relative autonomy, the research of the functionality is required to have a maximum of comfort, of security and effectiveness in its gestures. To put all the chances of cure on its side, it is important to be active, to stop smoking and to have a balanced food.

1 - Alimentation

To call into question its dietary habits passes by the fact of being ready to limit its consumption of foods or sweetened drinks (refined cereals, prepared fizzy drinks, biscuits, dishes, candies, processed products...), to think of eating local products, fresh vegetables (green and coloured) and the red fruits and blacks by avoiding cookings at high temperature (barbecue and cracklings), and to optimize the contributions in omega 3, trace elements, magnesium and vitamins C and D (anti pain and activator of the immune system)

The fodd without dairy produce and/or gluten-free can bring a comfort and a fall of the body disturbances.

To turn to a herb trade is a very interesting condition to relieve its evlls.

2 - Storage

Equipment

To avoid too low or too high storages preferably and to rather privilege storage with breast height.

To use mural wall cupboards with sliding drawers with facilitated opening and closing or wall cupboard with racks with low depth kind library (30 cm only) for free access without having to bend down to take an article at the bottom of the wall cupboard.

To buy a half-cupboard with shoes with reductions low depth (10 cm) very easy to use effortlessly to arrange its shoes.

To install a rehaussor with each settee or armchair, footboard, in order to bring a little height in articles which are low.

To use a scheme of 95 cm height work minimum in order to avoid forcing on all the top of the body (neck, shoulders, back).

To install a high table of bar in the kitchen which is used as service road, of and table work table of meal without having to bend down.

To choose chairs with comfortable assizes preferably high to avoid folding legs.

To make install toilets higher than the normal.

To use a shelf rather than a computer because the touch screen is functional. Hands

Kitchen ustensils

To buy ustensils with broad wrist to have the best taken.

To use ceramics knives whose blade is sharper.

To be accustomed to wrist with tools useful to piles such as can-opener, jar-opener, bottle-opener, corkscrew, mandoline, pepper mill and salt, potato peelers which are easy to use and especially which avoids forcing. The bottle-opener has been a companion of life for several years, just like the pile potato peeler which saves my force.

Useful breakage bulbs on sale in pharmacy facilitates the life.

To choose cleaning by disposable paper with the boxes of tissues to wipe or even the paper rollers with distributor.

To buy arrange-cups suspended to pose as regards work which is within reach of hands.

Chase

To make use of a caster bag (or caddie) to carry the races (no matter what difficult to carry too heavy on the level of the wrist and arm which support part of the weight. To choose a caddie with three casters in order to climb. To preferably carry the bags of race or another object with bags to broad wrists to relate around the wrists or on the front armlevers and even to the shoulders.

Cleaning

To use a brush vapor for the ground, the panes, the valves and fittings, the shower and the bath-tub, the wash-hand basin and the sink as well as a brush to vacuum-clean the ground with babywipe of single use and a small wrist for the furniture.

To use bottle shower gels pumps or better still soap.

To put on gloves of surgeon to wash the hair, to do the dishes or all other pieces of housework including in handling what protects the skin and decreases the sensitivity.

3 - Clothing

To privilege the leggings with sticking. Some, scraped inside for the winter which protect well from the cold.

To choose socks or low of application for blood circulation (to avoid sticking them difficult to put).

To buy hot gloves and softs out of silk (under-gloves) or wool

To privilege hot underwear specialized in the protection of the cold bound for the sensitive to cold people or in cold places (sticking, t-shirt, camisole...).

To choose clothing of color which affects the moral one. To leave the perenially fashionable black the winter to decorate warm colors or cold.

To remove the reinforcements in clothing (bra especially). To avoid the wearing of jewelry steel which is conductive electromagnetic waves. More the great attention must be carried to certain gold jewelry which can comprise an alloy of several also conducting metals of waves.

To privilege open shoes.

Not to use closings with loop neither laces neither boots to thread nor the flip-flops which are difficult to thread. Preferably, to take shoes with zipper no matter what difficult to wrist. The pumps are easy to use. The broken into white horses supple boots are very pleasant to carry even if they do not hold the foot well. Those out of acrylic resin are not hot and not tight. A sole inside can help to be hotter if the sole is not insulating enough ground. The dish is to be privileged or failing this, a small heel (4 cm maximum) preferably out of crepe which deadens the shocks and of the heels compensated for a better maintenance and to avoid the falls or imbalances.

Foot-warmers in the pockets isolate from the cold the hands and the feet. A fatty labial pomade for the lips avoids the cracks or cracks.

4 - Care of the body

A particular point can be planned in order to soften its disorders by care of the body: balneotherapy (antalgic effect and relaxing warm water, supports the muscular relaxation), massages two to three times per week at kinesitherapy and modellings.

Creams adapted to the body are difficult to find. The hospital proposes a preparation and a cream with the hyaluronic acid refunded by the social security. Certain bandages for the fingers are also refunded.

To use a feather bed rather than cloths and covers, easier of handling. In winter, the flannel fabric brings much heat or softness.

5 - Ergonomics with work

To buy thick pens or balls to be slipped around the pen, a pile stapler, fingerstalls rubber with barbs to sort paper, an arm of telephone, a shelf with casters, rest-elbows, gloves heating USB, a heating carpet, a small mouse, a rest-foot...

To think of putting on fine gloves out of silk.

6 - To develop its social network

To learn how to breathe deeply, practise a physical-activity, to take the air to oxygenate fabrics and to increase its rate of vitamin D, and to air themselves contribute to the greater comfort (for the physique and the moral one).

An aspect important not to neglect is to maintain the network of friends, the family and to have social activities, artistic or spiritual.

7 - Taking into account of the handicap

The law on the handicap of 2005 for the chance and equal rights, the participation and the citizenship of the handicapped people points out their basic rights and the obligation of solidarity of the whole of the company in their favour.

Constantly of work for disease during three years, the change on a station with forty kilometers of at home in 2009 caused six months a professional rupture (generated by additional tiredness and physical pains of the hands to all the top of the body). In parallel, I deposited a file of declaration of worker handicapped near the Département house of the handicapped people (MDPH) in order to obtain a priority of change. This recognition is useful also for the retirement, for the holiday vouchers (more advantageous refunding). It also makes it possible to profit from a third time for the examinations and competition and to constitute a file of service of the handicap for installation of its place of dwelling, its workplace and equipment or assistance to transport.

Installation of work station

Always given to improve my health, in September 2012, I deposit a file of installation of work station near my employer. The assault course begins then for the long ones and painful requests. The first obstacle consists in the difficulty in finding equipment adapted to my pathology. Second is to make coincide equivalent equipment, by three different suppliers, with the same rate. Third is to propose one trial period generally refused by the suppliers. Fourth is to recover coherent and right estimates by Internet within reasonable delays. The armchair and the rest-foot, lent gracefully during a week, were delivered to me, in September 2013, that is to say one year after my initial request then an office and a half-cupboard. In September 2014, I requested from my employer an in-depth study by an ergonomicist of the work which could refine my framework of work, to perceive my difficulties, to evaluate them and compensate for them by the recommendation of small equipment. The appropriateness of the purchase of a half-cupboard with small drawers with a ranking flat (kind architect) rather than the current use of large sorters of A4 format to broad back in a large cupboard appears judicious to me, just like a small mouse, heating gloves and a rest-wrist.

Right to compensation

The life plan of the person constitutes the right to the compensation of its handicap.

The service of the handicap financed by the territorial collectivities of the supply of a mural cupboard with drawers in the kitchen as well as small equipment of kitchen to piles such as can-opener, jar-openers, bottle-opener, pepper mill and salt, potato peeler and grater.

In addition, the installation of my shower room was financed by my financial backer with removal of a shower shoe of the Seventies for a shower with flat vat of ninety cm as well as the installation of tap with long nozzle at the various water supply points in the kitchen and the shower r

Disability

On the level of CPAM, three categories of disability to work exist following a stop in long illness.

8 - Various assistances

Human assistance

The mutual insurance companies even grant a human assistance to residence (household, chases, keeps of child) for one short period at the year. With my request, my mutual insurance company granted an exceptional assistance-housewife to me during several years. I could count on a regular support which saved me my energy and especially allowed a hygiene of my interior and incidentally a help the kitchen.

In parallel, I ordered my races by Internet in a supermarket close to my dwelling, with home delivery, in my kitchen. They was the first steps of the home delivery, before the "drive" created well by large commercial signs for the order by Internet and the delivery of the races in the trunk even of its car, with the store. What a relief!

The social security takes part in this service at the exit of hospital.

The social worker of staff helps the employees to assemble files and to propose any request for assistance.

The service of the pain of the hospitals targets speakers specialized in his relief (acupuncture, massages…) and offers the treatment appropriateness in the s

The moments of loneliness are large. I could compare them with the exit of maternity where the mother is exhausted of a maternity and a recent childbirth and which needs support, assistance domestic and culinary and temporary guard, somebody of reliable on which resting. A telephone call, a visit of friendship, one evening pizza, a fruit shopping cart, a hot dish, an exit movies organized, one afternoon" hammam", a baby-sitter, one transferred with the sea to take a fresh air...

All but not pity! This feeling which accentuates the discomfort and the taking into account of our entourage of gravity and the danger. The role of the entourage is consequently essential in order to leave insulation.

Material aid and financial

The installation of station perhaps facilitated by its employer through the funds for the insertion of the people handicapped in the civil service and the private sector.

The installation of the dwelling by the means of the service of compensation of handicap (PCH) within the Département house of the handicapped people (MDPH) after having deposited a file recognition of handicapped worker.

The AGEFIPH opens employment with the people handicapped in the construction of a community project, formation, adaptation to employment.

The employer, in his social aspect, brings a financial aid to their employees for a human help, and a material aid.

The social security can grant a financial aid on the expensive care, just like the mutual insurance company.

The cure at a watering-place is an asset to obtain more comfort. In Ald (affection long life), the cure is refunded. Rare are the people who are not relieved even partially.

The on-complementary offer of the services of refunding not to be neglected. Their subscription is annual and can be used on or more years if need be.

The request for long affection is made by the doctor for the fitness trail and the drugs related to the affection whose assumption of responsibility by CPAM allows refunding hundred percent.

An association of assistance to fibromyalgic was created. The fabric is rich useful information for the interested people.

Third part

The take-off

of the phoenix

I felt well that I had still something to learn on my disease. I did not resign myself to accept it. My will to go from before and to face it, to reduce it and reduce it to nothing was stronger than all. Not! I am not sick. It will not resist to me.

1.

On the way towards a better life

In September 2013, my energy to conquer my disease is always news. I turn to a speech therapist in order to improve my oral opening and the flexibility of my skin on my face. On the telephone, for an appointment management, the speech therapist indicates to me that I do not need it because my elocution is audible. She proposes to me to turn to a stomatologist who treats the neurological mouth and detections.

By chance, she advises me a stomatologist with eight kilometers of my place of dwelling. It has a long initial training. Its mission is the medical science of the oral cavity.

My first telephone making of contact with its dental assistant disconcerted me because the consultation was related to an oral panoramic radio so that the doctor can see with exactitude the origin of my evils.

I was persuaded that I did not have anything with the teeth. I went in the dentist since any young person and I was made look after my teeth regularly. I resigned myself all the same to do what is necessary because my curiosity and my will to advance pushed me in the action.

I thus find myself at the time of my first go in October 2013, in the end of the afternoon, I advance in a calm district. The assistant, a fair young woman of about forty year to the long hair dressed in raised white trousers of a white blouse and roadway of shoes introduces me into the white waiting room in which I am the only patient. She has the sharp glance and imposes by her only imposing presence a know-how. Pleasant and to listening, she explains me the cogency of the panoramic radio. I expect some surprises but certainly not with those imagined.

Then only, I observe intrigued the tables fixed on the wall. I am attracted first of all by a large horizontal table "dental Resonances" of Dr. Albert Roths on whom figure a panoramic photograph of the jaw with the correspondence of the teeth numbered with the body and their effect on health. Intrigued by this table which sits enthroned in bottom of waiting room, I read and try to decipher the significance in keeping with my teeth. Difficult analysis which leaves me at the same time perplexed and curious about comprehension because each tooth can be at the same time responsible for body symptoms and can also give an indication on psychological problems of the patient. For example, the tooth n° 35 corresponds to the algodystrophie of the shoulder and the muscular force.

Another table entitled Fibromyalgic "in search of its axes" explains the dysfunction of the axes of the human body on fibromyalgique in parallel with the normal posture. An imposing list of what feel that about which they complain, which depresses them and whqt obstructs them causes me shivers in the back.

Attentive with these indications, I cannot make a link reality since for me, on the one hand, my teeth are healthy because the visits in the dentist have been connected for my six years and on the other hand, my body is right and sufficiently stiff not to lean as on the mural image.

Over the years, the decays accumulated, the large amalgams and the crowns flowered in my mouth however maintained regularly by my dentist who, with each one of my visits, found a place to make turn his caster. I was consequently trustful on the diagnosis of the stomatologist who could not reproach me any dental anomaly on my teeth. My mouth was healthy.

None was lacking (except two torn off wisdom teeth former years).

However, I am with thousand places to imagine what will occur and revolutionize my life.

The doctor has been stomatologist and dental osteopath, for about thirty years.

Curious and in search of concrete explanations and of formations in order to make evolve its work, it has been interested in the fibromyalgia for several decades.

It accommodates me in a white big room of work decorated of large ficus close to the armchair of the patient and of its large wooden desk vis-a-vis the main door. It is large and thin, with the greying hair, of about fifty years. It gives to me a good impression in its white blouse of surgeon. He questions me on the reason of my arrival and consults my scanner thoroughly. Initially, he suspects a problem in my gums on the level of the incisors lower than the sight of a small cyst. Then he asks me to expose and borrow the long rectangular red carpet on the ground on two return tickets in order to see my approach. He informs me that my approach is dubious and that my basin is not right. He then proposes to me to be squatted. In front of my impossibility due to my muscular stiffnesses in all the muscles of the thighs and calves, of the arms and the back, it makes me lean ahead, tended legs and arms. Using one meter, it measures my major tended which is located at twenty-seven centimeters of the ground. Lastly, he asks me to bend down behind. I am carried out by bending the legs slightly. Not only, I cannot bend down, but in more I cannot catch up with myself if I fall because my hands prevent me from taking delivery of me flat because they are almost fixed with stiff and inflated fingers, reddened with the articulations of which impossibility of opening them completely and of closing them obsesses me the every day.

I observe his face and that of his collaborator whose stupor is let read easily. I have my problems but the fact of showing them puts to me quickly badly at ease, recognizing my weaknesses and my incapacities, at my age. I have explained being to him imprisoned in my body stiffened for eight long years and to have had the impression to have aged fifty years in a few hours! Ankylosed, my body seems to me stiff like a robot!

The doctor proposes to me to be installed on the armchair, observes and analyzes my mouth, manually touches the back of my neck on the level of the root of skull. Then, it makes a test in order to measure the galvanic current in my mouth. It puts to me "with the mass" by touching an amalgam with a ustensil. Without closing the mouth nor to swallow, I remake the preceding exercises on the carpet. My walk becomes heavier, more anchored in the ground, my rocker front gains twenty centimeters and with his assistance, I am able to squat me to two thirds. It is incredible! What did it make? That is worthy of a magician! My body does not answer in the same way any more. It gains in flexibility. I live again! It is the day and the night in a few seconds. I have the impression to have had a face lift and to feel me light like a feather. The doctor informs me that the effects are temporary at most of a few hours because the current in mouth mixed with saliva will induce an effect of stiffness proven. Indeed, the stiffness was reinstalled in the evening, blocking my neck and my shoulders ahead, in an unbearable vice.

But I leave grown this experiment because I have finally the hope of a better future. Optimist and full with enthusiasm, I start to dream of mobility.

I observe his face and that of his collaborator whose stupor is let read easily. I have my problems but the fact of showing them puts to me quickly badly at ease, recognizing my weaknesses and my incapacities, at my age. I have explained being to him imprisoned in my body stiffened for eight long years and to have had the impression to have aged fifty years in a few hours! Ankylosed, my body seems to me stiff like a robot!

My mouth is filled with mercury! Nothing astonishing that my health worsened. My body cannot about it support these important amounts of harmful foreign bodies any more. The fact is that the skeletal gimlet is obvious, the weight of my body ahead with plantar and dental supports thus modified. It is necessary and important to carry out its removal as soon as possible, in a slow way and specifies, according to a protocol concretized by an estimate validated by the two parts:

- two to three meetings of dental osteopathy not refunded by the social security in order to support occlusion. It is a question of if need be correcting the closing of the mouth by the fitment of the jaw without difficulty.-

The care will be long and expensive the more so as my mouth comprises about ten crowns and of old amalgams. After the care, my body will remain still charged with mercury which will be eliminated as month even a year. It is essential to daily drink two to three liters of water besides drinks annexes (tea, coffee...).

I ask him for explanations on the table of coincidence of the teeth with physical problems displayed in his waiting room. The doctor informs me that the teeth are in close relationship to the physiology of the body. They are in direct link with a body or vertebrae; the muscles of the jaws and those of the basin are of connection. So the not laterally balanced muscular tensions cause pains with the ankles, the knees, and the hips. It specifies the need for having a comprehensive view of the body and not of only one tooth to be looked after.

In addition, the amalgam (or leading) is the most used most known obturation and made up of an alloy of various metals including nearly fifty percent of mercury, thirty percent of money, thirty percent of copper and tin, as well as zinc, beryllium, zinc, money or palladium...) in order to improve qualities of the obturation. Its advantages are multiple energy of facility of handling, the speed of installation, with the great mechanical resistance and the good sealing on the long run as well as a weak cost with refunding by the social security in France.

But at the end of a few years, the negative effects on health cause the release of approximately fifty percent of the mercury in the mouth or in the bodies of the body (brain, kidney, liver, gastro-intestinal system).

This dysfunction is accentuated by the electro-galvanism which puts in presence two different metals in mouth with a liquid (amalgamates and crowns or prosthesis and saliva). Bacterial and viral infections or the disordered state of the immune system with the appearance of autoimmune diseases attack any healthy body. Only the demounting of the amalgams according to an adequate protocol with the patient is essential not to accentuate the harmful effects on the human body. Few experts launch out in the adventure. I was faithful to my dentist during thirty-five years, until his retirement. He never dared to try the experiment, pretexting the misdeeds of the intervention to the profit of their maintenance in mouth considering their seniority.

The finished consultation, I become aware with skepticism which my meeting is crucial and which it is the starting point towards a new life while interfering many interrogations with confidence that I have desire for giving to this unknown. But the experiment tries me considering the convincing result of this very first consultation.

Of return to my residence, I thought of the speech supported by the doctor. I wondered at the same time on the veracity of his statement and his competences. If all were true, the practice current and would be recognized government. I consulted his very explicit site which appears me to clearly emphasize its competences. It gives conferences, formations and even wrote a book on the subject.

I hesitated much to invest me in this process. The challenge is important: to recover my health. I put in the balance the number of years when the muscular frustrations, diminish, tensions and many daily impossibilities exasperate me as well as the real loss of almost ten years of my life in this yoke and especially the feeling to be old double of my age! The budget to be invested is dubious but consequent since the improvements will be noted progressively and the duration seems to be spread out over the year, even more. And to say that I thought of not having anything to look after in my mouth! What a revelation!

Rebith

My next appointment in November 2013 is intended to solve the big problems of imbalance occlusal of the osteopathic type. Using the caster, it is a question of helping my jaws to close themselves without embarrassment, and to release its side movements and of before behind and of rebalancing the supports of my jaw. The first reports are alarming. With the closing of my mouth, I do not have any possible movement ahead, behind, nor on the sides. My jaws are imprisoned one against the other without possibility of movement. I remember to have alerted my dentist in the years 1990 on this feeling right after having carried out a large amalgam. Its answer was like a chopper, refusing my report, with undoubtedly the feeling to failing this put its competences.

Some blows of caster later following targeted prints, my jaw is untied instantaneously. I then have the feeling pleasant to be released. At the same moment, a flood emerges in my calves, as a sharp torrent which circulates in my legs and my feet. I take again possession of my body.

It is enough to imagine happiness, the wellness, the hope found and comfort on the only use of the caster! I feel a lightness which I missed since so a long time. Two thirty minutes meetings each one were enough to come to end to these nuisances.

The next month, in December, comes it appointment at the stomatologist who transformed my life in a phenomenal way, unexpected and magic because the first go set the tone towards the revival, my resurrection and the hope towards a better life.

1 - Measurements of the galvanic current

The doctor measured the rate of galvanic current in each one of my teeth. Acceptable measurement is of less than 100 millivolts (mV) and less than 10 microamperes (my) per tooth. But my mouth presented this day of the incredible statistical data.

The teeth are numbered thus, from right to left on the jawbone: wisdom tooth 18 - molars (17 - 16) - premolars (15 - 14) - canine 13 - incisors (12 - 11 - 21 - 22) – canine 23 - premolars (24 - 25) – molar (26 - 27) - wisdom tooth 28 and mandible: wisdom tooth 48 - molars (47 - 46) - premolars (45 - 44) – canine 43 – incisors (42 - 41 - 31 - 32) - canine 33 - premolars (34 - 35) – molar (36 - 37) - wisdom tooth 38.

Jawbone: premolars: n° 15: 81 mV - n° 24: 143 mV- n° 25: 142 mV and molars: n° 16: 89 mV and n° 17: 76 mV - n° 26: 107 mV
Mandible: premolars: n° 35: 196 mV - n° 45: 200 mV - molars: n° 36: 131 mV - n° 37: 125 - n° 46: 215 mV - n° 47: 89 mV - wisdom tooth n° 38: 152 mV

2 - Probable origins of the fibromyalgia

I had made serious research on the evolution of the symptoms, the muscular ignition and the links with the dental care and my medical course through a detailed table.

I look like an obviousness the advance passed until the fibromyalgia: the catch of "tétracycline" at the three years age, my pregnancy, my two crowns posed with six and nine months after the birth of my daughter, the big intestinal problems just after the meal which followed, then my muscular ignition only five months after the installation of the last crown and three months after the vaccination of the DT polio.

I proves that after the birth of my daughter in October 2004, I consulted a dentist urgently (mine could not receive me) seven months afterwards for tooth aches in May 2005 which put a crown to me out of ceramics on the molar n° 46 after one work hour. I have the memory which it had of the evil to work, especially on the channels of my root all while being irritated. Then, two months afterwards, in July, another visit in another dentist of replacement ended in another ceramics crown on the premolar n° 35. In September of the same year, I am made vaccinate by my general practitioner of the DTP. Four months later, I suffer from generalized muscular ignition. Coincidences are striking in a few months of interval, no matter what a priori, without cause and effect link until my consultation of this famous December.

3 - Deposit amalgams

The stomatologist decides to begin the removal of the crown on the molar n° 46 — posed initially since eight years and half, then replaced in May 2005 by a dental mutual insurance company in 2008 (only three years afterwards) — whose intensity is very hight in millivolts. After having used the caster to cut out it, it extracts it from my mouth and poses on my chest. My neck comprises stiffnesses whose two points of pressure related to the fibromyalgia remain hard and painful. My arms are stiff when the doctor tries to position them to me one after the other behind my head. Muscular pains pull about me and prevent me from raising them behind my head. Then, it deposits it with its grip on the shelf of work, with fifty centimeters of my body. It practises new tests on my neck which is softened instantaneously. My arms pass behind my head without difficulty.

At the same moment, I then feel in my legs a strange phenomenon. Circulation is done naturally, a such torrent which runs in my calves and to my feet throughout all intervention. I have the feeling of a lightness. He then asks me to rise and go along his red carpet to see the phenomenon. After one moment of physical loss of reference mark, my body is seized again and my walk becomes surer, the feet anchored well in the ground. The doctor asks me to bend down ahead tended legs. I am carried out. Whereas my major tended had been with twenty-seven centimeters of the ground for eight years, they are found without any difficulty with seven centimeters of the ground. I do not return there! The muscles of my back, my thighs, my calves, my neck and my arms finally authorize me to lower me ahead. I note whereas my physical problem thus comes well from my teeth. No other explanation is possible. I regain the medical armchair and the doctor puts back the crown on my chest. My neck and my arms stiffen and my hands contract. He carries out the catch of print and poses a provisional tooth and appointment for another meeting gives me. I am filled of happiness. I am thus not sick! My health will thus improve of day in day as it indicated it to me.

Eight long years of monastic life, deprivations, physical preventions, fall of moral, concern... Eight years which prevented me living normally with my infant and from profiting fully, with impossibility of carrying it in my arms, of raising it, of running with or of lowering me, of making steps prolonged without muscular tensions on the calves, the shoulders and the neck, of playing the cards or any game of handling, of putting jewelry, etc. Eight years of smartness to lead or wash me, to cook and the acts domestic, to make my bed and to carry out to spare it and so much other difficulties. The tear with the eye, I start to dream of a better world. I dare to hope with the improvement of my life, my daily newspaper and with my future which is announced radiant. This day sounds the revival, my revenge on the life even if I must still wait a year or eighteen months even more still so that I eliminate the evil which corrodes my body without shouting station, which was propagated imperceptibly in my bodies to be reduced to the prison life, imprisoned in my ravaged body. I live again!

The doctor posed the crown to me fifteen days after because this period of time is essential so that the body is accustomed small-with-small and to thus avoid the physical nuisances caused by the precipitation of the care. However, four days were enough so that it breaks in my mouth with the pressure of food. It proves that I have an important allergy to zirconia and that I cannot have that special crowns "washed ultimate" and not "inlay core". The test was carried out by the doctor in his cabinet during my consultation and my body reacted instantaneously in the crispation accentuated (neck, arm and hands) with the accused crown. In possession of my new crown, the opening of my mouth is done larger. My colleagues pointed out to me to this period a clear improvement of my face rested and slackened with effect good mine. Number of enters asked for my secrecy of beauty to me! My skin was revitalized, nourished, coloured, dew and was alleviated, slackened with less oral wrinkles. I have had in addition, considering the circulation improved in my body, eliminated the polar hot underwear for this period and the layers superimposed from clothing in the top from the body (under-sweater, scarf or scarf, bonnet). My statute of extremely sensitive to cold woman was seen transformed.

In March 2014, new measures relating to the galvanic current are taken on which the current dropped appreciably as a whole after the two more important proportioned three months removal before:

Jawbone: premolars: n° 15: 78 mV - n° 24: 103 mV- n° 25: 63 mV and molars: n° 16: 85 mV and n° 17: 66 mV - n° 26: 93 mV

Mandible: molars: n° 36: 100 mV - n° 37: 101 - n° 47: 89 mV

The observation of the reduction in proportioning in mV is seizing on the remaining teeth. They are dependent enters by the galvanic current. The demounting of the most proportioned the influence inevitably downwards figures.

The molar n° 37 is filled with dental amalgam. The demounting of mercury under dental dam is essential. It is about a very thin and flexible latex square completely impermeable aiming to protection any intrusion of mercury by oral way in the vital bodies.

At the end of April, then the pulling up of my wisdom tooth arrives n° 38 which does not have during on the jaw opposite what can cause body disorders. It was neat on several occasions and comprises a large amalgam in its center and small on one of the edges. Pulling up was long and the cicatrization gave me pains during about fifteen days.

I can affirm that in spring 2014, of clear physical improvements make me find my energy and my dynamism. I also saw a strong attenuation of the nodules on my articulations. My arms are more mobile and can from now on function behind or in the air more easily. I find pleasant feelings of movements. Following the relaxation of the tensions and swellings, my front armlevers find flexibility. The feeling of wood end disappeared.

With demounting of crown n° 35 in June 2014 (posed initially in June 2005 whose intensity is very high in millivolts), still a revolution in my body is felt. I could note important phenomena of improvement such as the oral opening larger to four centimeters and half instead of two centimeters ten millimeters (with profit of two centimeters four millimeters), a strong attenuation of the nodules on my articulations (elbows, knees) and disappearance on the level as of ankles, my low-cheeks reinflated, a flexibility and a colouring of my skin with attenuation of the drought on the level as of hands and process of committed deflation of the tendons of the fingers, a better mobility in the possible stretching of the feet and toes and the correct nights eight hours of sleep. I have a feeling to live in the flexibility even if I am still stiff. I establish the obvious link of dental resonance on the body: the muscular force returns little by little thanks to this tooth (table of Dr. Roths) as if a clearing were on the way.

Then, the demounting of the amalgams continues during the summer, the crown n° 45 and the large amalgam on the tooth n° 47 improves little by little the unit of my disorders.

In July, with the tooth n° 45 (also strongly proportioned in millivolts): deposit crown and reconstitution of the piece of titanium tee core, my low-cheeks still gain in volume. Modelled face regains a suitable shape.

Since the summer 2004, I find the possibility of applauding. I intend the noise to strike it my hands one against the other with force, and flat. I in addition can, thanks to the deflation of the tendons of the phalanges close to the palm of the hands, to cross my fingers. Eight long years during which it was impossible for me to cross my fingers! That appears foolish but however this gesture did not make any more start from my daily newspaper. The only fact of thinking of it makes me cold in the back!

In September and October 2014, the crowns on the premolars 24 and the 25 are deposited then replaced.

At the dawn of the year 2015, the interventions with removals of the large amalgams of molars 15 and 16 follow one another then the spring of the 26 and 27. The gray color attenuated on my teeth (canine) which became whiter.

Most painful was the 27 because it is at the bottom of the mouth. My lips did not support any more the prolonged opening and them muscles burned me with the corner of the lips. The doctor had enormously difficulty working because it progressed almost blind. I was lengthened with horizontal on his armchair and positioned to him through managing to finalize his work which lasted one hour during.

I am grateful professionalism of the stomatologist, qualified and impassioned by his work which seeks to relieve the patient in spite of great difficulties according to its patients. I must pay him homage and well cordially thank it with his right value. It has worked for about thirty years so that its patients know the benefit of its diagnoses and its competences within the framework its work. I made a capital meeting in my life and I wish to transmit my enriching experiment which can get such a wellness that it would be egoistic not to disseminate the information with all.

Then, a crown steel (molar n° 36) always remains in mouth. However, three meetings of adjustments were necessary in five months. The doctor made the decision to replace it on the occasion because it seemed to him that it was not alleviating. To tell the truth, I felt as covered in mist, as in the "vaps", emptied, without promptness, constraint to advance without seeing the end of it, overworked by least work, with end before starting, without energy and power. As weeks, II felt in mouth an embarrassment developed. With each chewing, the food was captive and hung between two teeth. The opposite side had the same symptoms. It became difficult to eat easily. I was to take a toothpick to leave food their residences.

In December, the surprise was large during its removal. Mercury recovered my devitalized tooth! The specific procedure was adopted under dam. After the care, a provisional tooth was posed.

I left his cabinet with a vitality, an energy and a desire for doing one hundred meters! I am always astonished by the beneficial symptoms after my passage at the stomatologist. What a happiness to feel light! What a feeling of freedom!

I am always astonished by the instantaneous benefits received with each care. I rediscover with each meeting the surprise to feel important feelings inside my body and especially this flood in the legs. I arrive at knowing at which place the embarrassment is in the mouth for a small adjustment. I feel the aches to evolve. I am so much with the listening which I developed this competence. I am indeed one of the rare people who is hypersensitive.

What a pleasure of driving me more easily! What a joy of progressing and of gaining always more in flexibility! I left the meeting full with energy. I recovered to the writing from my book the evening even thorough by a supernatural force, a desire on the web for advancing and for finalizing my fixed goal and for concretizing the end of my course.

3.

All spread wings

Thirteen teeth deprived of harmful mercury and alloy for my human body gave again a blow of glare to dental enamel.

I do not have any more in mercury mouth from now on. However, my body still undergoes the misdeeds of this intoxication, of this poisoning in my bodies.

From day in day, I also gain in flexibility, my skin dew suffers less and less from drought, I find feelings forgotten since nearly one decade: to dry a sponge, to lower me, squat me, applaud, cross the fingers... and to even make some positions of yoga. My muscular force returns little by little even if I am still with fifty percent of the muscular capacities of a woman of my age. I make a rapid not on the regression of the fibromyalgia and I note with amazement that I do not have any more colitis, of distension, of rhinitis. Only some small isolated nodules are apparent on the left elbow and the right knee. Still resist of diminish with the hands and the legs and small morning cough from time to time.

The stomatologist brought a true body delivery to me. I gained seventy percent of physical benefit. It me gave again the taste to live, move, the desire for travelling, for living full-time, for sharing outputs with my daughter, for airing me, for making projects and for carrying them out, to give color to my life.

About fifty symptoms of the fibromyalgia from which I had suffered for eight long years, I am from now on with only one small ten in two years dental care. I can only note the dangerousness of mercury it human being in significant proportions and prejudicial. I already gained at least twenty years. I hope well to continue to reverse the process in the months to come. Time still will help with my improvement towards a flexibility increasingly more important thanks to the progressive evacuation of mercury within my bodies in all my body.

My account of life is summarized in this simple saying: "To make against all misfortune, good heart" because in spite of an unfavourable destiny, to accept what one cannot refuse, with courage no matter what it costs some and to seek to gain the best profit from it.

Fourth part

The fibromyalgia and the health expenditure

1.

Diagnosis of the fibromyalgia

or disease of chronic tiredness

The American college of rheumatology indexed in 1990 eighteen points of pressure on the body (on the basis of skull and neck, the articulations between the second coast and the sternum, the edges of the trapezius muscle, the internal edges of the scapulas, the upper parts of the buttocks, the elbows, hips and the interior of the knees. The diagnosis of fibromyalgia can be posed with eighty-eight percent if eleven of them painful and are tended.

However regarded a long time as a psychiatric disease, the fibromyalgia is recognized since 1992 by the World Health Organization (WHO) like a rheumatic disease.

The fibromyalgia is a disease which evolves and is reflected in the human body in a significant number of symptoms (nearly a hundred) whose principal ones are the fall of the physical performances (muscular fatigability, the tinnituses, allergy, disturbance of the intestinal transit time, eye trouble, of the sleep and mood, the stiffnesses morning, chronic general tiredness...), the fall of the intellectual performances and sensitivity to heat and the changes of temperature. Pains are added and a good amount of diminish which unbalance the axis of the body and accentuate this phenomenon. For certain people, the pains move on the body, when for others the migraine, chronic tiredness or the muscular contractions settle.

The most painful zones are close to the spinal column, generally the top of the body (the nape of the neck, the shoulders, the zone ranging between the two shoulders, the scapulas) and basin girdles it (low back, hips). Million people suffers from it in the world and do not know towards which to turn itself to decrease and especially stop this outburst of physical imbalances. Unfortunately, no biological sensor determines the origin of these evils.

The fibromyalgia understands three stages: the daily life is affected partially, pathology settles in a chronic way with night and diurnal intense pains and disturb the socio-professional relations, and the patient isolates himself.

Its release generally related to intense periods of is lived psychological painful or with food intolerances or heavy metals.

In France, three to five percent of the population are touched, of which the three quarter are women and generally in the neighbourhoods of forty.

The suffering is such as a help psychic and neurological is sometimes necessary: single solution to make less dramatic the health which is degraded without concrete explanation. The doctors generally engulf themselves in this medical and medicamentous way (analgesics, antidepressants) when the patient is tired even worn of this evil being. The person suffering from fibromyalgia (diagnosed or not) lives her evil being isolated, misunderstood and without support.

It is however enough to visualize the human body thus ravaged and to make the first observations by analyzing the walk of the patient: a shoulder is lower than the other and the hips start from the same side. The body is not any more in its axis and the posterior plantar supports are non-existent. Thus, all the weight of the body is rocked towards before skeleton. The back, the shoulders, the neck and the upper limbs and lower are thus solicited in an inadequate way and lose their reference marks, increasing imbalances and tensions.

In order to identify this disease, it is important to raise the good questions on its capacity with:

a) from a hygiene point of view of the house: to cook, Dishes with the hand, races, beds, the detergent out of machine, to pass the vacuum cleaner;

b) from a social point of view: to go to see friends or of the family, to drive a car, to climb, to make gardening, to go several hundred meters;

c) from a physical point of view: to have pains, to be tired, stiff, anxious, depressed.

The diagnosis of the fibromyalgia is simple because the answers are generally positive.

The fibromyalgia or disease of chronic tiredness is the disease of the century because it anaesthesia any activity of the human body. It makes each action physical difficult even impossible in a latent state of tiredness. It develops to touch innocent victims more and more. Many questionnaires of evaluation were set up as well as rating scales of the symptoms and pain.

A list indexes hundred symptoms of the fibromyalgia. The pain can be concretized in the form of aches, feeling stabs of burns or punctures, electric shocks, swarmings and the impression of muscular numbnesses.

2.

Financial expenses

The people suffering from fibromyalgia are expensive the company.

1 - Financial expenses for the company

The expenses engaged at parallel general practitioners, specialists and other medicines, sick leave, treatment and medical examinations... represent billion euros to the title of the French population.

At the level of one year, the international publications estimate at seven thousand euros per anybody the expenses engaged by the ministry for health.

This estimate is well below reality. The double would be more   suitable.
I had to call on the medical community in order to relieve my stiffnesses and to control my health status. I was well in spite of me a load for the company.

The declaration in affection long life (ALD) involves the full repayment of the expenditure engaged for the disease. The medical visits and care are refunded: kinesitherapy (1h30 per week), allopathy and homeopathy (every month), acupuncture (twice per month), dermatology, rheumatology, cure of care, occupational therapy with hospitalizations and medical examinations and biochemical and hematologic, VSL, pharmacy, social action of the social security, assistance-housewife, is a total of 14,000 euros rounded a year. The six months sick leave and the refunding of the dental care are added (4000 euros). The total load of the social security and the mutual insurance company is thus of 15,000 euros a year during ten years.

Then adjustment of station, housing, the service of compensation of the handicap, the social action employer, a total of expenditure rising with 16.OOO euros or 1.600 euros a year during ten years.

The overall costs of the State for my only person during ten years are 166,000 euros.

A complement of expenses to the sick load it in order to obtain a body comfort: osteopathy, hypnotizer, food supplements, balneotherapy, beauty products (creams for the body, the face and the hands)... of 1000 euros approximately a year and kinesiologist and care dental with 9,000 euros height are with my load a budget spent of 19,000 euros in ten years.

It is inevitable to multiply the integrality of these expenses by the number of years during which the disease prevailed.

In ten years, 185,000 euros were spent by the community to relieve my disorders of health.

2 - Funding

These large exceptional expenses engaged to improve my health inevitably burdened my budget. My projects of this fact were reduced to nothing.

 The body care is required to have a tiny comfort of life in a body of old woman. My dental expenditure was the object of minimal refundings on the basis of classical crown by the social security and my mutual insurance company to the amount of a hundred and eigty euros per tooth, supplemented by my complementary insurance to a total value of two hundred and forty seven euros per tooth to the amount of thousand five hundred euros for one year.

However, these expenses are the object neither of a whim of my share, nor of an aesthetic need but indeed for a vital need in order to stop poisoning with the mercury of which I was victim.

2.

If the secrecy were in your teeth?

The dental fibromyalgia of origin is a disease which should not exist. The exemption from payment of this evil related to mercury in mouth, prejudicial with the common run of people, is inadmissible for the patient. The organization east compels to swallow harmful quantities of toxic products however harmful for the environment. No benevolent glance stops this harmful and dangerous chain of use of mercury. The Superior council of public health of France (CSHPF) published a report in 1998 which gives information and recommends recommendations on the use of the amalgams.

In France, good information paper n° 261 (2000-2001) very provided on "the effects of heavy metals on the environment and the health" of Mr. Miquel made in the name of the Parliamentary office of evaluation of the technical scientific choices (deposited on April 5th, 2001 with the Senate) reveals in its second part of invaluable information on mercury in the dental amalgam. It was not followed of concrete facts nor of governmental decisional exceptional measures. However, its reading is rich lesson and discoveries on mercury and its misdeeds on health.

1 - Effects of the amalgam

Its paragraph C specifies the effects of the dental amalgam, material used to seal the dental fabric cavities affected by decays. Although also called leading, it does not comprise lead. It consists of liquid mercury (approximately one gram per amalgam) and other metalle powders some such as the money, copper, tin, zinc aiming at improving time of catch or the final mechanical properties of the mixture. The principal advantage of this alloy consists especially of a good sealing. Are added to that a perenniality in time, a facility of handling and a speed of installation, and a relatively weak cost.

The disadvantages of the amalgams are the hardness of the product, the unaesthetic one and the technique of specific station, and especially toxicity by the release of mercury and the electro oral galvanism. The electro galvanism is created by electric currents, of very low tension which are generated by the proximity of heterogeneous metallic materials. The oral cavity constitutes an organized different material puzzle (amalgams or different generation, alloys for prostheses and implants...), which generates various electric powers. They allow a release of metal ions which lead to the formation of a galvanic current (electric current of very low tension, studied by Galvani). He occurs a release of metal ions then when an amalgam is near other metals, in particular of an electropositive metal alloy, saliva playing the part of electrolysis then. Thus, certain scientists think that at the end of ten years, with the saliva and the chewing of food, two thirds of initial mercury are eliminated.

However an amalgam emits vapors of which a part is absorbed by the lungs. Mercury passes in blood, crosses the hemato-encephalic barrier, it is then trapped and accumulates in the brain. This mixture and the corrosion of the saliva with ions mercuric, of which a part seems to cross the wall of the small intestine and to accumulate in several bodies until oxidation and transformation into mercury salts to cause damage.

The composites for the small decays not allowing the effective obturation in the long run without warranty of sealing, the installation of amalgam Is privileged. Its multiplication in mouth is critical since it is known that the installation and the demounting of amalgams are two moments critical which are likely to increase brutally the mercury vapors just like the number of amalgams in mouth (threshold criticizes to seven).

A Canadian study recommends four amalgams for the adults, three for the teenagers, and for the children.

The information paper details the three types of consequences on health :

a) local reactions (allergies and the electro galvanism);

b) disorders and serious diseases: The toxicity of mercury is known: Neurologic disorders, neuromuscular or cardiovascular, nephretic, those on the phase of intra-uterine growth, the immune toxicity (the impact of mercury on immunizing defenses by modifying the intestinal flora, mercury would involve a sensitivity increased to the external aggressions and could make it resistant to antibiotics.)

c) and general consequences.

2 - Groups at the risks

It is also interested in the groups at the risks:

a) Pregnant women: By 1980, WHO recommended to limit the exposure of the women in age to have children. In France, this measurement made a double recommendation as well of CSHPF of May 19th, 1998 as of the Council about the dental surgeons. It is judicious to observe that this measure was adopted only after one deadline twenty years.

b) Other people at the risks: young children (chewing gum breast feeding and chewing), weakened adults (allergic and especially to the mercury or suffering of renal insufficiency) and adults with multi-decays.

c) Experts: The doctors stomatologists, dental surgeons, dental assistants are the first and most exposed to mercury of the amalgam. The exposure takes place at the time of the preparation, the installation, demounting, the recovery of the amalgams, and the polishing of the tooth, thus offering many occasions of direct contact and especially of mercury vapor inhalation. The mercury content in the air of the dentist's surgeries according to European studies tends to justify precautions and elementary measurements of hygiene know recapitulated by the CSHPF in its opinion of May 1th, 1998.

3 - Change of mentalities

En 2007, le mercure a été classé par l'OMS comme étant l'une des dix substances les plus toxiques avec l'arsenic, le plomb et l'amiante.

Since 2009, WHO recommends the progressive elimination of the products using of mercury, including the mercury amalgams. For as much, the organization estimates that a short-term total ban "would pose a problem for the public health and the dental sector".

The official position of our country is summarized in the report of the French Agency of public health of health products (AFSSAPS) of October 2005 which concludes with harmlessness from the amalgams

They are however prohibited in the countries of the north of Europe: Russia (1975) and Japan (1982), Sweden (1999), Norway then Denmark (2008). Several other European countries Austria and Germany followed the step.

Mercury is unanimously recognized nowadays like a very harmful substance for the human health and the environment.

It is in particular blamed in the multiplication of the "emergent diseases" (which multiply since the years 1980): fibromyalgia, allergies, depression, spasmophilia, migraines, diffuse pains, the Parkinson's disease, multiple sclerosis, autism... which could also be related to an intoxication with mercury.

The time between the latent intoxication at its beginning and the appearance of the symptoms can go up to fifteen years. Mercury is diffused slowly, durably throughout the intra-oral life, travels in our body on the whole of our bodies and poison seriously and silently the carriers of amalgams which absorb over one long life of negligible quantities of mercury.

According to a report published in 2012 by the European Commission, France uses a third of the fifty-five tons of mercury each year in the European Union for the realization of mercury amalgams. The international convention of

Minamata in October 2013 lays down a reduction in the use of the amalgams without to set constraints or objectives. The toxicity of mercury in the mercury amalgams continues to make debate.

4 - Questioning

How is it possible to accuse in France at the same time the mercury amalgams, their removal by a specialist (due to the mercury vapors), and their treatment like toxic wastes (tri in a special container), while preserving them in all impunity during decades in mouth, crossroads of the vital bodies (brain, lung, intestine)?

Would the danger on the environment be more prejudicial and worthy of interest for the government that its impact on the human body?

It is time to make change mentalities in particular into France and in all the European countries even on a world level which did not take yet the real measurement of the damage caused by mercury in the mercury amalgams on the Human one. The use of a highly toxic metal for dental care, probably at the origin of an intoxication and auto-immune disease estun medical scandal.

How can one then be still astonished by the emergence of new diseases and the development of certain autoimmune diseases? The precautionary principle or of prevention is not used for the people reached of the disease for a long time whereas the danger of mercury is perfectly known.

Not only the person suffers in her flesh from the ingurgitation from harmful products in all legality (antibiotic prescribes for young children to look after infantile diseases whereas it fragile the teeth in spite of the test laboratory not sufficient and the "tetracycline" is marketing without counter-indication or mercury in the mercury amalgams), then of the strong probability of which has occurred of an disease immune car without shouting station.

The feeling of imprisonment in the suffering and silence on the exemption from payment of this evil are particularly insupportable for the patients.

The divergence of opinions between country makes face with European resistance.

The State should not be any more one pit for the company which engages, with through the social security, to relieve and look after the innocent ones which will never cure harmfulness of mercury.

Measurements of prohibition of mercury in the amalgams are booked with some very minority countries in the European Union and with few countries overall in the world which have a responsible approach. They, by their action, saved part of their population at the same time as regards the human health, of the environment and a financial point of view.

Let us take as a model our neighbors who engaged in the responsibilisation of the wellness of their fellow-citizens. Let us guarantee that we will walk in their steps in the years to come.

Let us continue to dream at better days where the Human one is in the middle of the political scene.

Let us preserve our beautiful blue ground, all in roundness, protected from the misdeeds of the Man, by concrete conservative measures Our only will on a worldwide scale can leave with the future generations the ecological print essential to our planet.

We give means as of now and speak with one voice: our only force.

Conclusion

I wished this book in tribute to all these beings suffering in their flesh from fibromyalgia, which, by their courage and their immense force of life, certainly will be able to break the links which retain them captive and connected with the past. I give them the hope to find their youth too quickly lost.

I offer another glance on this disease. To leave the imprisonment of the suffering is not only one question of will but a goal to reach. Solutions exist.

I hope to have opened a window of hope and revival on the individual commitment in a combat of the every day in order to reappear a such phoenix.

Thanks

I wish to express all my gratitude and my deep respect with this helping hand guided by the professionalism and the convictions of the medical specialist stomatologist. Accompanied by its nice collaborator, they knew to punctuate the meetings of renewed notes of humour. I will never forget with which precaution and patience the care was lavished in my mouth between opened by the stiffnesses and especially this day of October 2013 when my life took another turning.

I have also a thought particular to the kinesiologist, the crossroads, which opened the doors of the creativity to me, and with the ergothérapeute who personalized his meetings towards the positive projection of consequent profits thanks to their professional competences and to their empathy.

Such an amount of good will to lead me towards a better and promising future, my dreamed becomes finally "reality".

***

I thank my parents also cordially: my mother, who believed in me and allowed to concretize my project, and my father whose star shines intensely in my heart and guides each one of my steps.

WHEAT OF THE MATTERS

List of works of the same author

Ebook, epub and delivers paper on plumissime.fr, Amazon.com, Fnac.fr and the booksellers

IN FRENCH

Adieu fibromyalgia ! Comment gagner 20 ans et retrouver une bonne santé
ISBN 979-10-95925-02-2

Petite étoile de Provence - novel - ISBN 979-10-95925-02-6

Au pays des Maharajahs - novel 8/12 ans - ISBN 979-10-95925-13-2

Sous l'Océan - Illustrated tale 8/12 ans - ISBN 979-10-95925-01-9

IN ENGLISH

Good-Bye fibromyalgia ! How to gain twenty years and to find a good health
ISBN 979-10-95925-17-0

Small star of Provence - ISBN 979-10-95925-29-3

With the country of the Maharajahs - ISBN 979-10-95925-32-3

Under the ocean - ISBN 979-10-95925-74-3

IN ITALIAN

Addio fibromialgia ! Come guadagnare 20 anni e trovare una buona salute
ISBN 979-10-95925-20-0

Piccola stella di Provenza - ISBN 979-10-95925-35-4

Al paese del Maharajahs - ISBN 979-10-95925-56-9

IN SPANISH

Adiós fibromyalgie! Cómo ganar 20 años y encontrar una buena salud
ISBN 979-10-95925-23-1

Pequeña estrella de Provence - ISBN 979-10-95925-38-5

Al país del Maharajahs - ISBN 979-10-95925-59-0

EN GERMAN

Lebewohl fibromyalgie ! Wie 20 Jahre zu gewinnen und eine gute Gesundheit wiederzufinden - ISBN 979-10-95925-26-2

Kleiner stem de Provence - ISBN 979-10-95925-41-5

Am Land Maharajahs - ISBN 979-10-95925-62-0

EN PORTUGUESE

Adeus fibromyalgie ! Como ganhar 20 anos e reencontrar uma boa saúde
ISBN 979-10-95925-53-8

Pequena estrella de Provença – ISBN 979-10-95925-44-6

Ao pais do Maharajahs - ISBN 979-10-95925-65-1

EN NETHERLANDER

Vaarwel fibromyalgie ! Hoe 20 jaar winnen en een goede gezondheid terugvinden - ISBN 979-10-95925-50-7

Kleine ster van Provence - ISBN 979-10-95925-47-7

Aan het land van Maharajahs –ISBN 979-10-95925-68-2

Illustrations of cover : Fotolia – evgeniya_m

and Photographer Alberto Gray - Châteauneuf-du-Pape

Printed in USA by Amazon

Completed to print in september 2016

Legal deposit : september 2016

Les Éditions Plum'issime

15 boulevard Limbert B- 84000 Avignon
plumissime.fr   plumissime123@gmail.com

Find all news of Laurence Estienne of www.plumissime.fr
www.facebook.com/Laurence.estienne.Auteur/

N° ISBN 979-10-95925-17-0

© Laurence Estienne, 2015 All rights reserved

This one does not authorize, at the end of the article L122-5-2° and 3°a, on the one hand that copies or reproductions strictly booked with the private use of the copyist and not intended for a collective use and on the other hand analysts and short quotations in a goal of examples and illustrations – Any representation or reproduction integral or partial made without the assent of the author or his having cause I illicit – L222-4 article.

This representation or reproduction, by some process that it either would thus constitute a counterfeit sanctioned by the L.355-2 articles and following of the code of the intellectual property.